Hair Care Formulas
to make you
Look Your Best

by

PHILLIPE COKER

Hair is a protein filament that grows from follicles found in the dermis. Hair is one of the defining characteristics of mammals. The human body, apart from areas of glabrous skin, is covered in follicles which produce thick terminal and fine vellus hair. This is a simple introduction about the human hair. However, in this book we want to let the readers understand how to maintain and look after their hair properly. The ability to look after your hair properly stems from your understanding of, first, the types of hair. Generally, it is my intention to help you make you look as gorgeous as you can be with your hair (either your natural hair or artificial hair).

What is a natural hair?

"Natural hair" typically refers to hair that has not been chemically altered with relaxers, perms, or straightening treatments. It is the hair that grows naturally from the scalp without any artificial interventions to change its texture or structure.

"Artificial hair" on the other hand refers to synthetic hair, which is a man-made material designed to resemble and mimic the appearance of natural human hair. There are various types of artificial or synthetic hair used for different purposes. Here are some common categories:

Synthetic Hair Extensions:

These are often used to add length, volume, or color to natural hair. Synthetic extensions are made from artificial fibers, such as polyester or Kanekalon, and are available in various textures and styles.

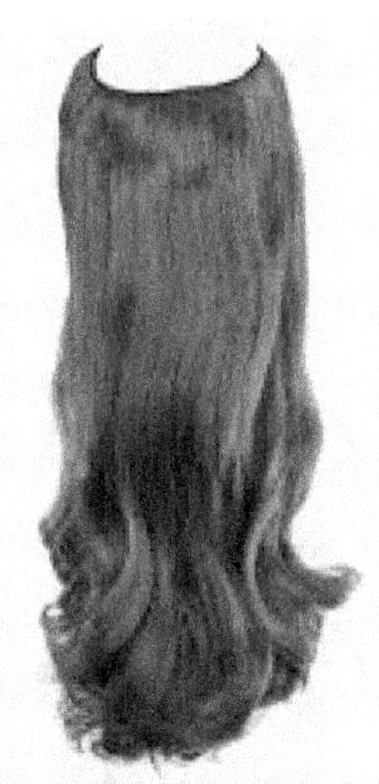

Wigs:

Synthetic wigs are popular for those looking to change their hairstyle temporarily or experiment with different looks. They come in a wide range of styles, colors, and textures. Some high-quality synthetic wigs closely resemble natural hair.

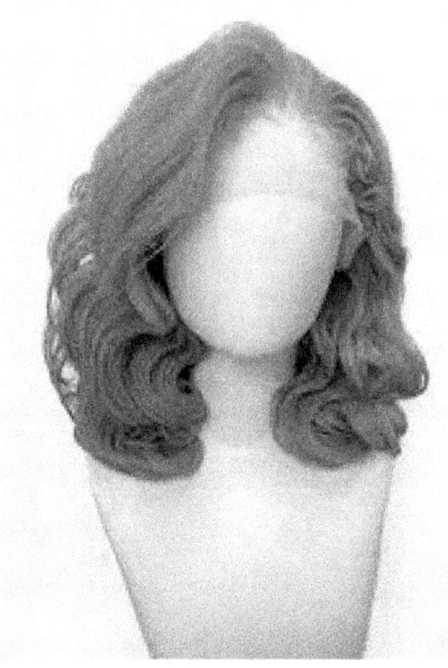

Clip-In Hair Pieces:

These are small sections of synthetic hair attached to clips. They are convenient for adding highlights, volume, or length to specific areas of the hair without a long-term commitment.

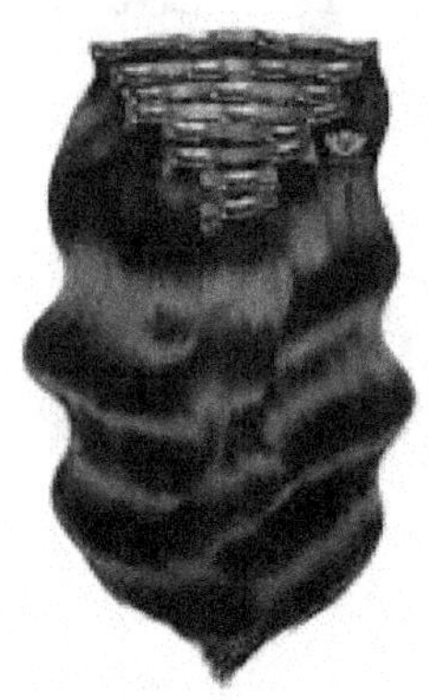

Ponytail Extensions:

Synthetic ponytail extensions are designed to be attached to the natural hair to create a longer or fuller ponytail. They are quick and easy to use for an instant hairstyle change.

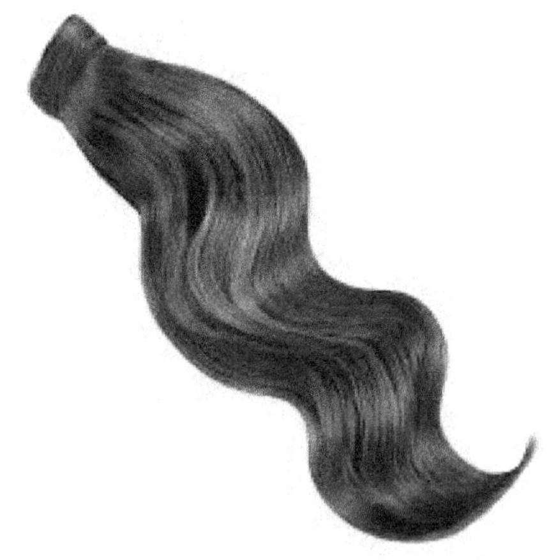

Braiding Hair:

Synthetic hair is commonly used for braiding styles, such as box braids, Senegalese twists, and cornrows. It is often lightweight, making it easier to create intricate styles.

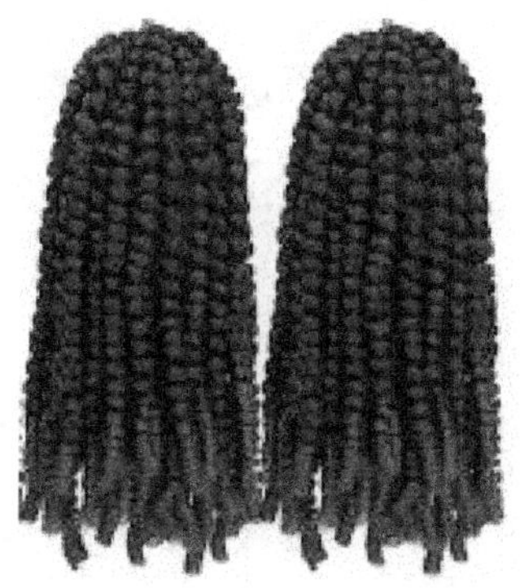

Toy and Costume Wigs:

Synthetic hair is frequently used in wigs for costumes, theatrical performances, and events. These wigs can be styled in various ways and come in vibrant colors and unique textures.

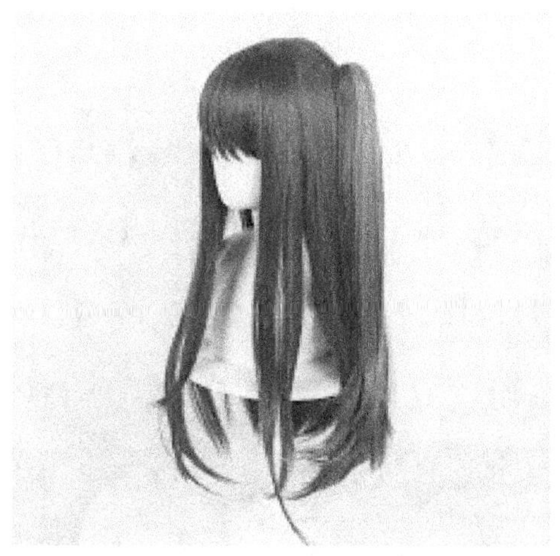

I

What we discussed previously is just a very brief insight on natural hairs and artificial hairs. What I want to achieve in this book is to help ladies look as gorgeous and beautiful as possible whether they are on their natural hair or on their artificial hair. For us to achieve that, we need to understand basic concepts like hair treatment and the rest. But first of all, we need to look at the hair types. There are different hair types, and for you to take care of your hair properly you need to identify your own hair type. This is because the different hair types have different methods or ways of maintenance or treatment. It also helps you understand what kind of enhancement to add to your hair, that is for those who wish to add some more touches to it. That said, let us look at the hair types we have.

Several hairdressers prefer categorizing hair shapes into four distinct groups: straight, wavy, curly, coily. However, in the field of medicine and scientific research, this classification system is not used by scientists. Now, why exactly do we have different hair types? Of course there is an explanation. The existence of different hair types is primarily due to genetic and evolutionary factors. Human hair varies in texture, thickness, and curl pattern, and these differences are largely influenced by genetic inheritance and adaptation to environmental conditions. Let's see some reasons why there are different hair types:

1. **Adaptation to climate:** Human populations have evolved in diverse climates, ranging from hot and humid to cold and arid. The different hair types observed today can be attributed to adaptations to these environments. For example, tightly coiled hair (kinky) may provide protection against the sun in hot climates, while straight hair might be more advantageous in colder regions.

2. **Genetic diversity:** Genetic factors play a significant role in determining hair type. Different populations around the world have unique genetic backgrounds that influence hair characteristics. Families and ethnic groups often share similar hair types due to the inheritance of specific genes.

3. **Hair follicle shape:** The shape of the hair follicle largely determines the curl pattern of the hair. Round hair follicles tend to produce straight hair, while oval or elliptical follicles contribute to curly or coily hair. This shape is determined genetically and varies among individuals and populations.

4. **Adaptation to sunlight:** The density and texture of hair can influence how much sunlight reaches the scalp. Straight hair may allow more sunlight to reach the scalp, which could be beneficial in regions with less sunlight. In contrast, coiled or curly hair may provide more protection from the sun.

5. **Cultural and social influences:** Cultural and social factors have also played a role in shaping perceptions of beauty and influencing hair practices. Different cultural norms and preferences have led to the creation and maintenance of diverse hairstyles and hair care practices.

There could be some other reasons why we have different hair types, but everything culminates to evolution and genetic factors. The characteristics of hair that were advantageous for survival and reproduction in different environments were passed down through generations. Let us now take a look at the four different hair types.

STRAIGHT HAIR

Characteristics

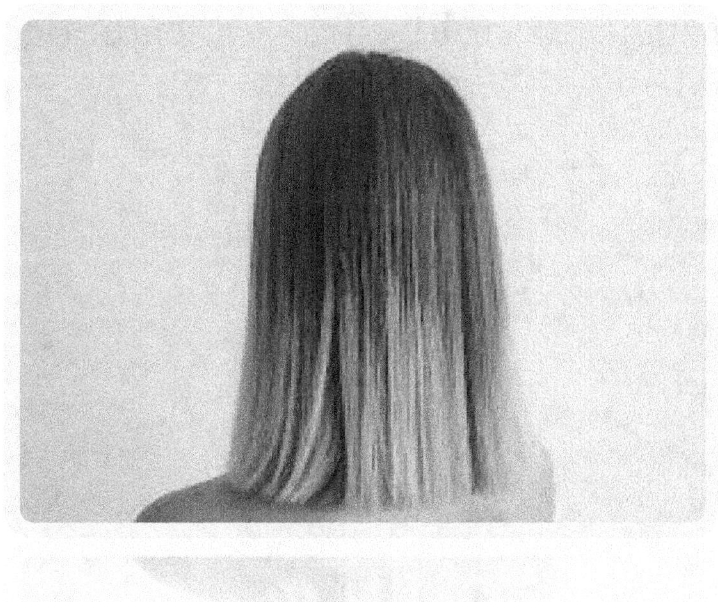

- Straight hair typically has a smooth and sleek texture.
- The hair shaft is round, which allows for a straight appearance.
- It reflects light well, giving it a shiny appearance.
- It tends to be more prone to oiliness at the scalp due to the direct path of natural oils.

Straight hair is often easy to style and can hold sleek looks well. It may lack volume compared to other hair types.

CHALLENGES

- Straight hair may struggle to hold curls for extended periods.

WAVY HAIR

Characteristics

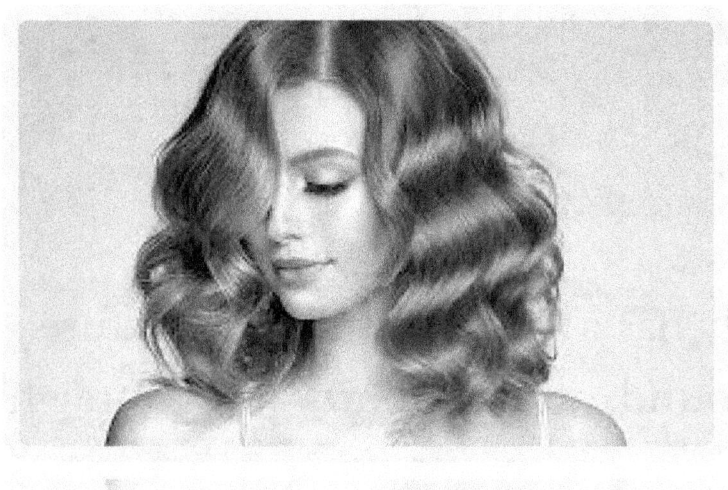

- Wavy hair falls between straight and curly, forming an "S" pattern.
- It has a thicker texture than straight hair.
- The hair shaft is usually oval, contributing to its wavy appearance.

STYLING

- Wavy hair can be versatile, allowing for both straight and curly styles.
- It may have more volume and hold curls better than straight hair.

CHALLENGES

- Wavy hair can be prone to frizz, especially in humid conditions.

CURLY HAIR

Characteristics

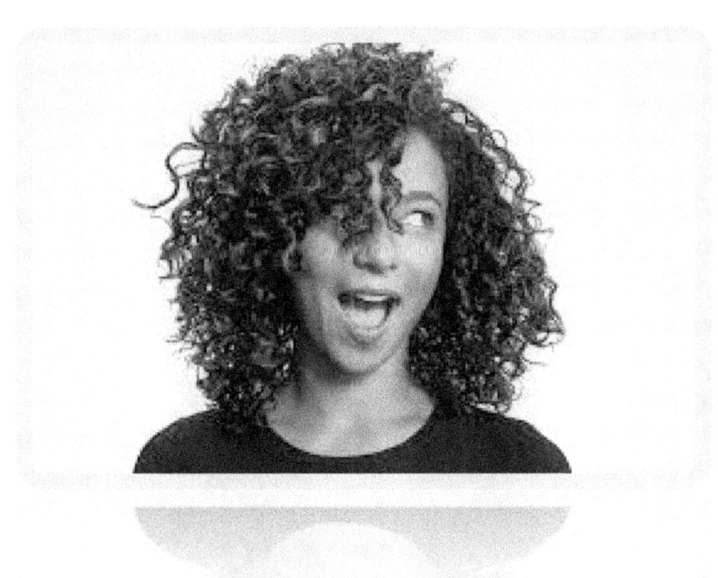

- Curly hair forms spiral or ringlet patterns.
- The hair shaft is often oval or elliptical.
- It can range from loose curls to tight coils.

STYLING

- Curly hair can hold curls well and offers versatility in styling.
- It tends to be more prone to dryness due to the natural oils having a harder time reaching the ends.

CHALLENGES

- Managing frizz and maintaining moisture balance can be common challenges.

COILY (KINKY) HAIR

Characteristics

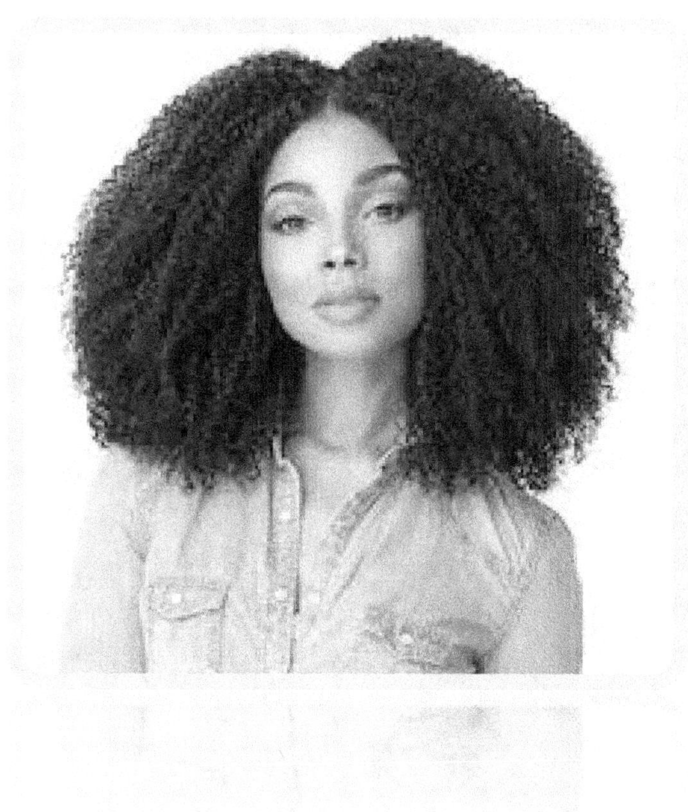

- Coily hair has a tight curl pattern, forming tight coils or zig-zag shapes.
- The hair shaft is often flat or ribbon-like.
- It may have a dense and voluminous appearance.

STYLING

- Coily hair is highly versatile for different styles, including braids and twists.
- It can experience shrinkage, appearing shorter than its actual length.

CHALLENGES

- Coily hair may be more prone to tangling and can require careful detangling practices.
- It may be more susceptible to dryness, requiring consistent moisturizing.

II

We have looked at what I will call "basic knowledge" of the different hair types that we have, in the previous chapter: straight, wavy, curly and kinky. Which of these is your hair type? It is important that you identify your hair type before you continue reading this book.

Now that you have identified your hair type, let us go ahead and show the various ways we can use to make us look beautiful and gorgeous in a natural way. This includes hair treatment, maintenance and care. It also includes the basic act of washing the hair at home. Every hair type has a care routine peculiar to only it, and we are going to outline them. Hair enhancement is also made much easier here because you are now aware of your hair type. In the previous chapter, we treated some challenges we face with the different hair types. Several enhancement methods have been developed to make up for the problems or loopholes one may face if you have a particular hair type. For example, curly hair tends to be prone to frizz. To minimize frizz, avoid towel-drying vigorously; instead, use a microfiber or cotton T-shirt to gently squeeze excess water from the hair. That said, enhancement can be achieved via the use of different enhancement creams, or just naturally;

with nothing. Now we are going to take each of these hair types and look at how to care for them and enhance them where necessary.

Note: The term "hair enhancement" can refer to both artificial and natural methods, depending on the context.

I.   STRAIGHT HAIR

Maintaining and caring for straight hair involves a combination of proper washing, conditioning, styling, and protection. Here are some tips to help you keep your straight hair healthy and looking its best:

Washing:

Sulfate-free Shampoo: Sulfates are detergents that can strip the hair of its natural oils, leading to dryness and frizz. Choose a sulfate-free shampoo to gently cleanse your hair without causing excessive dryness.

Washing Frequency: Straight hair tends to show oil more quickly than other hair types. Washing frequency depends on your scalp's oil production and personal preference.

Some people may need to wash daily, while others can go a few days between washes.

Conditioning:

Use a Suitable Conditioner: Choose a conditioner that matches your hair type and concerns. For straight hair, a lightweight, hydrating conditioner is often sufficient. Apply it mainly to the ends, where the hair is older and more prone to damage.

Deep Conditioning: Regular deep conditioning treatments help maintain moisture balance and prevent dryness. Use a deep conditioner or hair mask once a week to provide extra nourishment.

Drying:

Air-drying: Allowing your hair to air-dry whenever possible helps minimize heat damage. If you need to use a hair dryer, use a low-heat setting to reduce the risk of damage.

Towel-Drying Technique: Pat your hair dry with a microfiber or soft cotton towel instead of rubbing vigorously, as rough drying can lead to frizz and breakage.

Brushing:

Wide-Tooth Comb: Use a wide-tooth comb to detangle your hair, starting from the tips and working your way up to the roots. This helps prevent unnecessary breakage.

Avoid Brushing Wet Hair: Wet hair is more prone to breakage, so wait until your hair is damp or mostly dry before brushing.

Styling:

Heat Protectant: Apply a heat protectant spray or serum before using heat styling tools to minimize damage from flat irons, curling irons, and hair dryers.

Appropriate Styling Products: Choose styling products designed for straight hair, such as smoothing serums or anti-frizz creams. These products can help control frizz and add shine.

Trimming:

Regular Trims: Schedule regular trims every 6-8 weeks to prevent split ends and maintain a neat, healthy appearance. Trimming also promotes overall hair health.

Protecting at Night:

Silk or Satin Pillowcase: These materials reduce friction, preventing tangling and reducing breakage. They also help maintain your hairstyle for longer.

Loose Tying: If you have long hair, loosely tie it in a low ponytail or braid before bed to prevent knots and tangles.

Avoiding Excessive Manipulation:

Limit Styling: Excessive use of styling tools can lead to damage over time. Try not to style your hair every day, allowing it to rest and recover.

Gentle Treatment: Treat your hair with care to avoid breakage and split ends. Avoid tight hairstyles that can cause stress on the hair shaft.

STRAIGHT HAIR ENHANCEMENT

If you want to enhance the beauty of your straight hair and achieve a polished and sleek look, there are various techniques and styling options you can consider. Here are some enhancement techniques for straight hair:

STRAIGHTENING TECHNIQUE: Straightening your hair involves using heat styling tools to transform your natural texture into a straight, smooth, and sleek look. The most common tool for straightening hair is a flat iron, but blow-drying with a round brush can also achieve straight results. Here's a more detailed explanation of each technique:

1. Flat Iron Straightening:
   - Preparation: Start with clean, dry hair. Apply a heat protectant spray or serum to safeguard your hair from heat damage.

- Sectioning: Divide your hair into manageable sections using clips or hair ties. Smaller sections allow for more precise straightening.
- Temperature Setting: Adjust the flat iron to the appropriate temperature for your hair type. Lower temperatures are suitable for fine or damaged hair, while higher temperatures may be needed for thicker or coarser hair.

Straightening Process:

- Take a small section of hair (about 1-2 inches wide) and place the flat iron close to the roots.
- Gently glide the flat iron down the hair shaft in a smooth and controlled motion.
- Repeat this process section by section until all of your hair is straightened.

BLOW-DRYING WITH A ROUND BRUSH:

- Preparation: Begin with clean, damp hair. Apply a heat protectant or smoothing serum to protect your hair from heat.

- Sectioning: Divide your hair into sections using clips or hair ties to make the blow-drying process more manageable.

Round Brush Technique:

- Take a small section of hair and place the round brush underneath it.
- Use the blow dryer with a concentrator nozzle to direct the airflow down the hair shaft while simultaneously brushing through the section with the round brush.
- Repeat this process, working through each section until your entire head is dry and straightened.

TIPS FOR SUCCESSFUL STRAIGHTENING

- Proper Heat Protection: Always use a heat protectant product before applying heat to your hair to minimize the risk of damage.
- Even Sectioning: Divide your hair into small, even sections to ensure that each part is straightened thoroughly.

- Consistent Motion: Whether using a flat iron or blow dryer with a round brush, maintain a steady and controlled motion to achieve a smooth result.
- Temperature Awareness: Adjust the heat settings based on your hair type, and avoid excessive heat to prevent damage.
- Quality Tools: Invest in high-quality flat irons or blow dryers to ensure even heat distribution and consistent results.

III

WAVY HAIR

Wavy hair has a texture that falls between straight and curly, offering a unique set of challenges and opportunities. Proper care and maintenance can enhance the natural beauty of wavy hair, providing definition and minimizing frizz. Here's a guide to care for and maintain wavy hair:

1. Shampoo and Conditioning:
- Hydration: Use a hydrating, sulfate-free shampoo to prevent wavy hair from becoming dry and frizzy. Sulfate-free formulas are gentler on the hair and help retain natural oils.
- Conditioning: Apply a moisturizing conditioner to keep wavy hair hydrated and manageable. Focus on the mid-lengths to ends, where wavy hair tends to be drier.

2. Detangling:

- Wide-Tooth Comb: Detangle wavy hair with a wide-tooth comb, starting from the tips and working your way up. This helps prevent breakage and minimizes disruption to natural waves.

3. Washing Frequency:
- Balanced Washing: Wavy hair tends to be prone to dryness, so find a balance in washing frequency. Washing too often can strip natural oils, while too infrequent washing may lead to product buildup.

4. Styling Products:
- Curl Enhancers: Use curl-enhancing products, such as mousses or creams, to define and enhance the natural waves. Apply these products to damp hair, distributing them evenly for consistent results.
- Anti-Frizz Serum: Wavy hair can be prone to frizz, especially in humid conditions. Apply an anti-frizz serum to control frizz and add shine.

5. Drying Techniques:

- Air-Drying: Let wavy hair air-dry whenever possible to maintain its natural texture. Gently scrunch the hair while it dries to enhance the waves.
- Diffuser Attachment: If using a hairdryer, attach a diffuser to help evenly distribute airflow and enhance the natural waves without causing frizz.

6. Haircuts for Wavy Hair:

- Layered Cut: Consider a layered haircut to add movement and definition to wavy hair. Layers can help prevent the hair from becoming weighed down and enhance the natural wave pattern.
- Long Bob (Lob): A lob is a versatile and stylish option that complements wavy hair by providing a manageable length with movement.

7. Protective Styles:

- Loose Braids or Twists: For overnight styling or when you want to protect your waves, consider loose braids or twists to prevent tangling and breakage.

8. Nighttime Care:

- Silk or Satin Pillowcase: Use a silk or satin pillowcase to reduce friction, preventing frizz and maintaining the integrity of your waves.

9. Deep Conditioning:
- Weekly Treatments: Treat wavy hair to a deep conditioning treatment once a week to replenish moisture and keep it healthy.

10.   Avoiding Excessive Heat:
- Limit Heat Styling: Reduce the use of heat styling tools to prevent damage. Embrace your natural waves and reserve heat styling for special occasions.

WAVY HAIR ENHANCEMENT

Enhancing wavy hair involves bringing out the natural wave pattern, adding definition, and minimizing frizz. Here are some tips and techniques to enhance the beauty of wavy hair:

1. Curl-enhancing Products:

- Mousse: Apply a curl-enhancing mousse to damp hair, distributing it evenly. Mousse helps define waves and adds volume without weighing the hair down.
- Curl Cream: Use a curl-defining cream to enhance the natural texture of wavy hair. Apply the cream from mid-lengths to ends for optimal definition.

2. Scrunching Technique:

- Gentle Scrunching: After applying styling products, gently scrunch your hair using your hands. This technique helps encourage the natural wave pattern and adds texture.

3. Diffusing:

- Use a Diffuser Attachment: When blow-drying wavy hair, attach a diffuser to the hairdryer. The diffuser helps distribute heat evenly and enhances the natural waves without causing frizz. Use a low-heat setting to minimize damage.

4. Plopping Method:

- Plopping: Plopping is a technique that involves wrapping wet hair in a T-shirt or microfiber towel to enhance curls and reduce frizz. Leave the hair wrapped for a period of time (typically 15-30 minutes) and allow it to air-dry or use a diffuser afterward.

5. Twisting Sections:

- Twist Strands of Hair: Twist small sections of damp hair around your fingers to enhance and define the waves. This method can be done while the hair is drying or as a styling technique.

6. Braiding:

- Loose Braids: Create loose braids before bedtime to wake up with enhanced waves. The braids add texture and definition to wavy hair without using heat.

7. Layered Haircut:

- Consult with a Stylist: Consider getting a layered haircut to add movement and definition to wavy hair. Layers can prevent the hair from becoming weighed down and enhance the natural wave pattern.

8. Sea Salt Spray:

- Natural Texture Enhancement: Use a sea salt spray to enhance the natural texture of wavy hair. Spritz it on damp hair and scrunch for a beachy, tousled look.

9. Avoiding Heavy Products:
- Lightweight Formulas: Opt for lightweight styling products that enhance waves without weighing down the hair. Heavy products may flatten waves and contribute to limpness.

10.   Regular Trims:
- Prevent Split Ends: Schedule regular trims to maintain the health of wavy hair and prevent split ends. Healthy hair holds a style better.

11.   Overnight Styles:
- Bun or Loose Twists: Create a loose bun or twists before bedtime to wake up with enhanced waves. This is a heat-free way to style wavy hair.

12.   Protective Styles:

- Protect Hair While Sleeping: Use a silk or satin pillowcase to reduce friction and prevent frizz while you sleep.

IV

CURLY HAIR

Curly hair is prone to dryness, frizz, and tangling, and hence requires special attention. Because curly hair often gets dry and frizzy, we need to be careful with how we treat it to keep it looking great. The plan is to make sure our curls stay healthy, well-cared-for, and looking their natural best. We'll talk about how to keep them hydrated, handle them gently, and use the right products to make those curls pop. Whether your curls are loose or tight, we'll go through some easy tips to keep your hair feeling good and looking awesome.

1. Washing:
- Sulfate-Free Shampoo: Use a sulfate-free shampoo to prevent stripping natural oils, which can lead to dryness. Curly hair tends to be drier, and sulfates can exacerbate this.
- Co-Washing: Consider co-washing (using conditioner only) between regular shampoos to maintain moisture without over-cleansing.

2. Conditioning:

- Hydrating Conditioner: Choose a rich and hydrating conditioner specifically designed for curly hair. Apply it generously, focusing on the mid-lengths and ends.
- Deep Conditioning: Use a deep conditioning treatment or hair mask regularly to provide extra moisture and enhance curl definition.

3. Drying:

- Air-Drying: Allow your hair to air-dry whenever possible to minimize heat damage. Gently scrunch your curls while drying to encourage their natural shape.
- Microfiber Towel or T-Shirt: Use a microfiber towel or a soft cotton T-shirt to gently squeeze excess water from your hair without causing frizz.

4. Detangling:

- Wide-Tooth Comb or Fingers: Detangle your hair when it's wet using a wide-tooth comb or your fingers. Start from the ends and work your way up to avoid breakage.

5. Styling:

- Leave-In Conditioner: Apply a leave-in conditioner to keep your curls hydrated and defined. It helps reduce frizz and adds a protective layer to your hair.
- Curl Defining Products: Use styling products like curl enhancers, gels, or creams designed for curly hair to define and hold your curls in place.

6. Trimming:

- Regular Trims: Schedule regular trims every 6-8 weeks to prevent split ends and maintain the shape of your curls. Curly hair tends to be more prone to breakage, and regular trims promote healthier growth.

7. Protecting at Night:

- Silk or Satin Pillowcase: Use a silk or satin pillowcase to reduce friction, preventing frizz and tangles. Alternatively, you can use a silk or satin hair wrap or bonnet.

8. Avoiding Excessive Manipulation:

- Hands Off: Once you've styled your hair, avoid touching it too much to prevent disrupting the curl pattern and causing frizz.
- Low-Manipulation Styles: Opt for protective hairstyles like braids or twists to minimize daily manipulation.

9. Product Buildup:

- Clarifying Shampoo: Periodically use a clarifying shampoo to remove product buildup from your hair, which can weigh down curls and affect their definition.

10.   Humidity Control:

- Anti-Humidity Products: In humid weather, use anti-humidity products to help control frizz and maintain your curly style.

CURLY HAIR ENHANCEMENT

Curly hair enhancement involves employing specific techniques and practices to emphasize and define the natural curls, waves, or coils present in the hair. Curly hair often requires special care to minimize frizz and showcase its inherent beauty. Here are some suggestions for enhancing curly hair:

1. Prioritize Hydration:
- Choose Moisturizing Products: Opt for sulfate-free shampoos and conditioners with moisturizing properties to keep curly hair well-hydrated and reduce frizz.
- Regular Deep Conditioning: Incorporate routine deep conditioning treatments to supply additional moisture, sustaining the health and vitality of your curls.

2. Select Appropriate Styling Products:
- Curl-Enhancing Formulas: Invest in styling products tailored for curly hair, like curl creams, gels, or mousses. These products define curls and provide hold without weighing down the hair.
- Use Leave-In Conditioner: Apply a leave-in conditioner to damp hair for ongoing moisture retention and enhanced curl definition.

3. Opt for Suitable Haircuts:

- Curly-Optimized Cuts: Choose haircuts that complement your unique curl pattern. Layered cuts can prevent a pyramid shape, while well-defined layers accentuate natural movement and bounce.
- Consider Dry Haircuts: Explore the option of getting haircuts when your hair is dry, allowing the stylist to customize the cut based on your natural curl pattern.

4. Adopt Gentle Drying Techniques:

- Air-Drying: Permit your hair to air-dry to reduce heat damage. To boost curls, scrunch your hair upward while drying to encourage natural curl formation.
- Use a Diffuser: If utilizing a hair dryer, employ a diffuser attachment to evenly distribute heat, enhancing curls without inducing frizz.

5. Explore Protective Styles:

- Pineappling at Night: Before bedtime, gather your curls at the crown of your head and secure them loosely with a satin or silk scrunchie to preserve curls and minimize friction during sleep.

- Experiment with Braids or Twists: These styles can define curls once unraveled.

6. Utilize Curl-Enhancing Tools:
- Finger Coiling: Define individual curls by wrapping small sections of hair around your finger.
- Incorporate a Denman Brush: Use a Denman brush for detangling and defining curls during styling.

7. Regular Trims for Maintenance:
- Trim Split Ends: Schedule regular trims to eliminate split ends, promoting the overall health of your curls and preventing breakage.

8. DIY Hydrating Treatments:
- Homemade Masks: Create DIY hydrating hair masks using ingredients like avocado, honey, or yogurt to add moisture and nourishment to your curls.

V

KINKY HAIR

Kinky hair, often associated with tight curls or coils, has unique care and maintenance needs. This hair type tends to be more prone to dryness and requires special attention to retain moisture and definition. Here are some tips for caring and maintaining kinky hair:

1. Gentle Cleansing:
- Sulfate-Free Shampoo: Use sulfate-free or low-sulfate shampoos to prevent excessive dryness. Consider co-washing (using conditioner to cleanse) between regular shampoos to retain moisture.

2. Deep Conditioning:
- Regular Deep Conditioning: Kinky hair thrives on moisture. Deep condition regularly to provide intense hydration, strengthen the hair, and enhance elasticity. Use a deep conditioner or hair mask at least once a week.

3. Moisturizing:

- Leave-In Conditioner: Apply a leave-in conditioner or moisturizer to damp hair to keep it hydrated throughout the day. Focus on the ends and areas prone to dryness.
- Water Spritzing: Keep a water and glycerin mixture in a spray bottle to refresh and moisturize your hair when needed.

4. Protective Styling:

- Braids, Twists, or Bantu Knots: Protective styles help minimize manipulation and protect the ends of the hair. These styles also retain moisture and promote hair health.
- Wigs or Weaves: Using wigs or weaves can be a protective styling option, allowing your natural hair to rest and grow.

5. Detangling:

- Finger Detangling: Use your fingers to gently detangle your hair, starting from the tips and working your way up. This minimizes breakage and preserves curl definition.

- Wide-Tooth Comb: If needed, use a wide-tooth comb for detangling, especially when applying conditioner.

6. Low-Manipulation Styling:
- Avoid Excessive Styling: Limit the use of heat styling tools to prevent heat damage. Embrace your natural texture and opt for low-manipulation styles to maintain curl pattern.

7. Nighttime Care:
- Satin or Silk Bonnet/Pillowcase: Protect your hair while sleeping by using a satin or silk bonnet or sleeping on a satin or silk pillowcase. This reduces friction and prevents breakage.

8. Trimming:
- Regular Trims: Schedule regular trims to remove split ends and maintain the overall health of your hair. This helps prevent breakage and promotes growth.

9. Use Natural Oils:

- Sealing with Oils: Apply natural oils like jojoba, coconut, or olive oil to seal moisture into your hair after applying leave-in conditioner. These oils also add shine and improve manageability.

10. Avoid Harsh Chemicals:

- Limit Chemical Treatments: Minimize the use of harsh chemicals and relaxers, as they can lead to damage and breakage. Embrace your natural texture and consider protective styles instead.

KINKY HAIR ENHANCEMENT

Kinky hair enhancement refers to various techniques and practices aimed at maximizing the natural beauty, texture, and health of kinky hair. Kinky hair is characterized by tight curls or coils, and enhancement involves methods to define and accentuate these natural patterns. The goal is to promote curl definition, minimize frizz, and maintain overall hair health. Here are some specific aspects of kinky hair enhancement:

1. Moisture Retention:
- Deep Conditioning: Regular deep conditioning treatments are crucial for moisturizing and nourishing kinky hair. Deep conditioners with rich ingredients like shea butter, coconut oil, and other hydrating elements help combat dryness.
- Leave-In Conditioners: Apply leave-in conditioners to damp hair to lock in moisture and provide continuous hydration.

2. Curl Definition Techniques:
- Twist Outs and Braid Outs: Twist or braid the hair to define curls and coils. After allowing the twists or braids to set and dry, unravel them for well-defined, textured curls.
- Bantu Knots: Create small Bantu knots to enhance curl definition. Allow the knots to dry and then unravel them for a defined and textured look.

3. Styling Products for Kinky Hair:
- Curl Enhancing Products: Use styling products specifically designed for kinky hair, such as curl

creams, gels, or styling puddings. These products help define curls, reduce frizz, and provide hold.

- Natural Oils: Apply natural oils like jojoba, olive, or coconut oil to seal moisture and add shine. These oils also aid in preventing breakage.

4. Protective Styling:

- Braids, Twists, or Locs: Protective styles help minimize manipulation, reduce breakage, and protect the ends of kinky hair. These styles also retain moisture and promote hair health.
- Wigs or Weaves: Using wigs or weaves can be a protective styling option, allowing the natural hair to rest and grow.

5. Stretching Techniques:

- Banding or African Threading: Stretch kinky hair without heat by using banding or African threading techniques. This helps reduce shrinkage and showcase the length of the curls.

6. Trimming and Haircuts:

- Regular Trims: Regular trimming helps maintain the health of kinky hair by removing split ends and preventing breakage.
- Shape Enhancing Haircuts: Consider haircuts that enhance the shape of your natural curls, such as layers or shaping the hair to frame the face.

7. Avoiding Heat Damage:

- Limited Heat Styling: Minimize the use of heat styling tools to prevent heat damage. If heat is necessary, use a low-heat setting and apply a heat protectant.

8. DIY Natural Hair Treatments:

- Homemade Masks: Create homemade hair masks using natural ingredients like avocado, honey, and yogurt to provide extra nourishment and moisture.